# First Aid Book

# Role of First Aid, Training and Disciplines, Initial First Aid Steps, Equipment, First Aid Skills and Its Safety Measures

# Table of contents

## Introduction

I want to thank and congratulate you for downloading the book, "First Aid Book: Role of First Aid, Training and Disciplines, Initial First Aid Steps, Equipment, First Aid Skills and Its Safety Measures,"

This book contains information about first, the role of first aid, its training and disciplines, equipment and the basic skills to handling various conditions .The book also contains safety measures as you carry out a first aid. This ensures you own safe even as you help a victim.

The language used in writing this book is easy to understand. You will be gifted with the knowledge on handling various emergency issues even without going to a first aid class.

Thanks again for downloading this book, I hope you enjoy it

## Chapter 1: First Aid and Its Role

First aid is assistance given to someone that has suffered from an immediate illness, condition, emergency, so as alleviate a condition, preserve a life or treatment to a condition.

It can also be referred to as an intervention before the help from a medical professional. Some of these actions include performing a Cardio-Pulmonary Resuscitation or a complete treatment to minor injuries like applying of plasters to a cut.

A first aid is done as you wait for the arrival of an ambulance or a health professional to a scene of the emergency.

First Aid is normally performed by a layperson. This is mainly a person trained in providing basic levels of a first aid. You can also do it if you have some knowledge and basics about it. For mental health purposes medical practitioners have come up with mental health first aid, an extension of a typical first aid.

There is a variety of situations that require first aid. A number of countries have come up with regulations that specify the level of first aid you can provide for a circumstance.

You, therefore, require special training and equipment in your environment you are operating from, at gatherings, at school, in your car, etc.

First aid does not require specific equipment or its knowledge; there are a number of improvisations one can come up with to save a life. Many people that perform a first aid are not trained in even the basics.

## The Role of a First Aid

Life will not be perfect for you every day, accidents exist, and, therefore, first aid should be a tool in our lives. A first aid will prevent further injury, promote a recovery and preserve life.

Wherever you will be, there is an accident, and you need to rise up and save a life. You should not be a helpless witness. A situation can be worse and having basic knowledge of first aid will save somebody.

First aid is the first thing that always needs to happen to a victim of a condition or illness. You as a lay person well be required to provide the assistance until the medics arrive.

This chapter will bring to the light the significance of a first aid. The knowledge about first aid will help in emergency situations. In a case like a poisonous gas inhalation, heart problems and other critical health conditions you will become even useful to the medics when they arrive.

First aid will ensure appropriate methods of medical administration are provided to a victim. Basic information like the brain taking 6 minutes before it expires from lack of oxygen will help.

With first aid, you can also help yourself. A lay person is also a human being and, therefore, can experience the accidents in life. With this knowledge at a workplace will help save you and those you work with.

You have discovered that first aid knowledge is important, but it also should be a necessary requirement for some people like day care staff and nannies. A life guard should also be certified in first aid procedures.

In business, you also need the basic of first aid. The extent of first aid training will depend on some specifics of a place of work. In case you work in a high-risk environment, you need the basic first aid knowledge. Some of these places include machine shops, factories, and industrial plants. Some employers offer their staff with basic first aid training.

A proper first aid should be carried out so that a condition does not worsen. You need to be keen, careful and not time wasting.

## Chapter 2: First Aid Disciplines and training

First aid training is divided into a number of disciplines. The disciplines of training are mainly the areas of work or a condition to be handled.

Below is a discussion of some of the first aid training disciplines you need to know:

Mental health first aid: This is an independent type of first aid training different from the typical first aid. This kind of first aid training dwells on mental health situations. The knowledge of this kind of first aid training enables you identify primordial signs of a mental health victim and give appropriate guidance.

Oxygen first aid: Here one is equipped with the knowledge of providing oxygen to casualties suffering from conditions that result in hypoxia.

Aquatic or Marine first aid: This kind of first aid training is normally practiced by professionals in a water environment. They are equipped with the knowledge to help after water-based accidents. Some of the professionals include divers, lifeguards, and mariners.

Battlefield first aid: This training equips you with the knowledge in dealing with the wounded in armed conflicts.

Hyperbaric first aid: This discipline of training will enable deal with SCUBA diving emergencies like bends.

Wilderness first aid: This disciplines trains you on dealing with conditions whereby emergency responders have delayed. This can be as a result of the location of that place, the weather, equipment availability. The knowledge will enable you handle a condition for a number of hours or even days.

A first aid manual is not enough when it comes to hand-on training. The training will also vary in various regions. In this chapter, you will get to learn about the various programs offered in each region. There are a number of societies and organizations that offer for first aid. Some of them include:

The Lifesaving Society: LSS in Canada provides first aid for life guards and the public,

The Red Cross: A leading first aid training organization all over the world

St. John Ambulance: Is another well-renowned organization that offers advanced first aid courses all over the world.

The Canadian Ski Patrol in N. America is an organization that provides first aid training for ski patrollers and the public. Also in Canada there is the Heart and Stroke Foundation.

Other programs are corporate training programs which provide their own special training.

Some ambulances and fire services offer basic first aid courses to the interested people; you can reach them through their Emergency Contacts.

Other programs include the British Red Cross a part of the worldwide organization that provides commercial and personal first aid training.

For higher levels of training, you can go for training as a:

Paramedic: This is a most qualified and professional for ambulance personnel. The paramedic has a range of specialized drugs and items like intubation kits. It is rare to find someone that has achieved a paramedic level.

First Responder: This is often aimed at professionals like police officers; a lay person can also become a first responder for assistance in emergencies before the arrival of an ambulance.

Emergency Medical Technician (EMT): This is the most prominent; many people are qualified to this level of first aid training. If advanced some of the training include resuscitation, spinal care, and patient handling.

In some countries, people obtain their training through voluntary organizations or private training.

# Chapter 3: Initial Action Steps in a First Aid

This is well defined by the famous mnemonic "Go DR SHAVPU." A first aid should first thin of their safety before approaching a victim. The mnemonic refers to Gloves On for GO, Danger for D, R for responsiveness, S for Scene Clues, History for H, and assessment to for response of the victim in the place of AVPU.

The first and paramount aspect of a first aid is your own safety. You should not place yourself in danger; a victim cannot help a victim. Make sure you safeguard yourself first as you assess the situation; begin the treatment after taking these steps.

As you get to a scene put on personal protective equipment. The most pronounced is the impermeable glove. Be conscious of gas leaks, live electrics, fires and falling objects even after protecting yourself with protective equipment. There are also human factors to be conscious about. Some of them include uncooperativeness, bystanders and aggressors at a scene. Always involve the police so as to enable control the scene if these situations appear. For uncontrollable situations stay clear and call emergency medical services.

When approaching a scene, there are a number of things to pay attention to and even asking questions about.

Some of the questions include what could have happened. Have a mental picture of an incident and try a treatment for the victim.

Assessing the scene includes knowing the place of incident, what might have the incident, get some history from the witnesses and how long ago the incident happened. Ask all these as you continue with the treatment.

Be sure to listen. As you operate on the victim, you may overhear the witnesses talk. This can help in your first aid. Note what is said since you may not get time to interview a witness.

After ensuring your safety, pay attention to the victim's response. There are a number of initial responsiveness checks you can carry out. You can look at the victim and read the responses from speech to body signs and facials. This can tell if the victim is alert.

You can assess the victim using the AVPU scale that stands for Alert, Voice, Pain, and Unresponsive. Spontaneous looks by the victim shows are termed as alertness. Some of the indicators include

The eyes: they open spontaneously, look around and even appear to see you calculate the alertness of the victim.

The Response to voice: the victim replies, understands, obeys commands like open your eyes or look at me.

If the victim isn't alert but responds to voice, you can say they are voice responsive.

Pain means any physical stimuli. A stimulus can be a tap, a shoulder shake, sternal rub; getting your knuckle to a sternum, breastbone or between nipples. Other stimuli include the nail bed squeeze on victim's finger using a flat edged object, ear lobe squeeze using your thumb or forefinger to hard squeeze a victim's ear. Responses like groaning and any movement shows a response to pain. The AVPs show the extent of a patient's consciousness. If the victim is not alert, you should call for professional like ambulance or an emergency service for assistance.

In the case whereby the response is to voice and pain, use a recovery position to help secure them. If a victim does not respond to voice and pain, they are unresponsive, and you must urgently perform more checks on their critical life systems like key life critical airways, breathing, and circulations. (ABCs)

## Chapter 4: Equipment for First Aid

Equipment for first aid will depend on condition, personal protection, and medication purpose. This chapter will give you knowledge on equipment for a number of conditions that need to be handled.

### a) Condition equipment

The first conditions are trauma injuries. Some of these injuries include burns, bleeding and bone fractures. Their equipment is mostly found in the first aid kit. The equipment includes dressings and bandages.

Bandages are normally known as adhesive bandages include sticking plasters. The sticking plasters can be shaped for a particular part of a knuckle. Moleskin is the equipment used for treatment and prevention of blisters.

Bandages always secure the wound. They do not need to be sterile you can use it on a plaster.

Dressings for first aid are sterile and work for wounds. More dressings include sterile eye pads, gauze pads, non-adherent pads with a non-stick Teflon layer and petrolatum gauze pads (airtight dressing for sucking chest wounds.

Other types of bandages include gauze roller bandages which are breathable, absorbent and even elastic.

Elastic and pressure bandages are used for sprains. Elastic roller bandages also Vet wrap are effective pressure bandages, durable and waterproof.

Triangular bandages are another type of bandage commonly used as slings, to tie splints.

Other equipment includes butterfly closure strips working as stitches for closing wounds in the case of higher response. These strips seal infection in unclean wounds.

To clean wounds, the first aid kit also contains the saline, soap when it comes to superficial wounds once bleeding has ceased.

To deal with infections in abrasions and around wounds antiseptic wipes and sprays are a good solution.

The sterile pad is usually soaked in cooling gel in the case of burn wounds before dressing.

The adhesive tapes uses are always hypoallergenic.

For clotting issues especial in armed grounds like the military, hemostatic agents are used when one has severe bleeding.

## b) Personal Protection Equipment (PPE)

Protective equipment will help you against any risks as you help the victim. One of the risks includes infection. Some of the common PPEs include gloves which are used once and disposed to avoid cross infection and goggles for eye protection.

Surgical masks to help reduce the risk of airborne infection. They can be used on the patient at times. A mask used by the patient should not have an exhale valve.

Tweezers are used for removing splinters, trauma shears for general use and cloth cutting, scissors and lighters for sanitizing the pliers and tweezers.

Alcohol pads are good for sanitizing equipment and dressing broken skin, irrigation syringe are used for cleaning wounds with sterile water. The stream of liquid will flush out dirt and debris.

Other equipment include the a source of light, an instant acting cold pack, alcohol rub or hand sanitizer, a thermometer, an emergency blanket, penlight, cotton wool for applying antiseptic lotions, cotton swabs and safety pins.

### c) Medication equipment

This is rare in public cases but can be witnessed in personal, family or home first aid kits. The type of medicine depends on scope of practice. The medication is mainly life saving. The kit is assigned for laypersons for the public or employees. They include pain killers and relief medicines.

In the case of life-saving the medication used includes Aspirin. Aspirin mainly serves as a medication for chest pain.

For wilderness use and summer camps, an Epinephrine Auto-Injector is used to temporarily reduce airway swelling for an anaphylactic shock.

Epinephrine does not treat anaphylactic shock but only opens an airway to prevent suffocation giving time for the arrival of other treatments. Its effects are short-lived, and the swelling of a throat may return. This medication, therefore, requires an accompaniment with other drugs until it works. Some of the medications include intubation.

Diphenhydramine branded Benadryl can treat and prevent anaphylactic shock. In emergencies, it advised that non-solid drugs be taken rather than tablets and capsules.

In the case of pain killers, Paracetamol is the most common pain-killing medication. It can be a tablet or syrup.

To treat sprains and strains anti-inflammatory painkillers like Ibuprofen and NSAIDs can be used. Anti-diarrheal Codeine can also be used as a painkiller.

For symptomatic relief, anti-diarrhea medication like Loperamide can be used. This is very paramount in those areas where dehydration caused by diarrhea kills children.

Other treatments include oral rehydration salts and antihistamine.

In the case of poison treatments practices like taking activated charcoal, use of emetics to induce vomit and smelling salts like Ammonium Carbonate can help.

# Chapter 5: Basic First Aid Handling Skills

The first conditions are the **ABCs**. These include the Airway, the breathing, and the Compressions also known as primary assessments.

An airway is a significant part of the human body. The first aid for an airway condition is simply a head-tilt-chin-lift. This act opens the airway effectively and safely.

This is the first part checked before carrying out a first aid. This is an entrance and exit of oxygen and carbon dioxide respectively. If an airway gets blocked and left unhandled, it may result in a cardiac arrest.

When doing a "head-tilt-chin-lift" technique

- The victim should be lying on their back also known as supine.
- One hand should be on the forehead and the other under the chin
- Tilt the victim's head backward and have the chin lifted.
- The victim's jaw line should be perpendicular to the ground.
- A conscious victim normally maintains an open airway, can be talking and their airway is adequate
- You can also check for the visibility of the mouth and get rid of obstructions that removable with a finger

**Breathing first aid:** When a victim has stopped breathing, the respiration can be restored by insufflations; breathing air into their body cavity, the victim may also experience a cardiac arrest.

Call an ambulance the moment you realize the patient is unconscious. To check for the breathing;

- Open the patient's airway and place your cheek 3 to 5 cm away from the victim's mouth
- Also gently place your palm on center of the victim's and detect the signs of breathing

The signs of breathing may include:

1. Feeling the airflow on your cheek
2. Hearing the airflow at the side of your face
3. Notice the rise and fall of the chest
4. Smell the victim's breathe
5. Under your hand feel the victim's chest rise and fall

Always provide rescue breaths for respiratory arrest victims. If you cannot detect the breath, then start a CPR. Protect yourself using a CPR mask Start by giving two rescue breaths.

You can perform this by maintaining an open airway using the head-tilt-chin-lift, plugging the nose with your free hand, in an airtight manner put your mouth on victim's mouth and gently blow air that can make the chest rise and allow it to exit before giving another breathe as you do the CPR compressions.

**Compression first aid:** This first aid enables blood flow and gaseous exchange to be restored in a victim and even leave the victim conscious. This is done by squeezing the heart in the victim's chest.

Compressions can be performed regardless of the victim. A compression is normally performed on the victim's sternum or breastbone.

In adults, 8 years and above a palm is placed in the center of the chest; between a nipple the nipple line for adult females. Depending on the size of the breast you can also use two palms with fingers interlocked to locate the line. Have your shoulders directly above your hands and have your arms straight. Push down firmly depressing the chest to about a third of its depth

In children, place a palm in the center of the chest just between the nipples and bring your shoulder just above your hand, with your arm straight, and perform the normal compression with a single arm.

For infants less than a year, use a fore and a middle finger. Have the forefinger at the center of child's chest and the middle just below in on the chest compress normally using the arm's strength.

First aid for bleeding, the bleeding could be external and internal bleeding. External bleeding can include abrasions, excoriation, laceration, incision, and a puncture wound. Noticing an external bleeding is usually easy since blood is seen, but the source might be the problem. Also check the backs and other hidden parts for the wounds.

The primary techniques for dealing with bleeding include Rest, Elevation, and Direct pressure. The rest enables the healing process easier since the wound is not experiencing any disturbance.

Elevation works for the periphery body parts like the head and limbs. Here you need to raise the part as high as you can, and you can use furniture or anything that holds the part high. For a leg lie on your back and raise the leg.

Direct pressure will involve using the hand to exert pressure on a minor injury. You need to elevate your hand just above the heart and press arm to slow the pressure. The flow reduces; the bleeding reduces and the clotting is assisted.

Once you have dealt with the bleeding, dress the wound. You should use a low-adherent and sterile pad. This does not stick to the wound but absorbs the blood coming from it. The dressing should be tight on the arm and apply some direct pressure. The check for this is by raising your arm just above the chest and pressing a finger. If a pink color on the finger does not appear in two seconds then the dressing is too tight and if bleeding gets back then apply addressing and don't interrupt the saturated one which holds the clots.

**Nose bleeding first aid**: pinch the soft part of the nose firmly between thumb and a forefinger, you can do this by yourself or the victim by themselves.

The victim should lean the head slightly forward and breathe through the mouth. Avoid tilting the head back to avoid ingesting the blood which may cause vomiting or choking. If you are unable to stop the bleeding after 10 minutes of direct pressure, assess your blood flow. Use an ice pack on the ice bridge to stem the blood flow. If the condition persists, seek medical assistance.

If an object was embedded in a wound, don't directly remove it. Press around the object using the sterile gauze. For a gun wound, puncture or stab do the ABC assessments and call for an ambulance. Sit the victim to allow the heart function as effective as possible or lean the patient to the injured side keeping the healthy side from invasion attack. In the case of an amputation, do an ABC and call for the medics.

**For internal bleeding**, blood leaks from inside. This can cause pain and shock and cannot cause blood loss. This kind of breathing requires immediate attention as it may easily cause death. Some of its causes include vehicle accidents, falls, gunshot wounds, explosions, stabs, and surgery.

Some of the signs of an internal bleeding include blood from mouth or nose, a clear fluid from the ear, blood in stool, blood in urine, blood in vomit, blood from birth canal or pregnancy, chest bruise, pain on vital organs and fractured femur.

The bleeding may not appear if you see any signs of shock and no injuries suspect internal bleeding. Check for changes in skin color. In cases of internal bleeding, the skin may become cold and pale.

**First aid for heart attack and angina**, heart attack is caused by the deprivation of oxygen to the heart muscles. This condition mostly occurs when at rest and less rare after exercise. An angina is a less severe heart attack due to a small blockage. Angina mostly occurs after strenuous exercise or long periods of stress. Angina alleviates after a period of rest whereas a heart attack does not get relieved even with a rest.

Some of the symptoms of a heart attack include chest pain; tightness in chest, nausea and indigestion, pale skin, grey skin, an impending sense of doom and denial.

These conditions mostly have a medication; could be pills or a spray. The victim should always administer their medication by themselves. You can only remove the lid of their medicine to avoid getting a migraine headache. Both medications are administered below the tongue. If the patient cannot do the medicine by themselves, you need to call for an ambulance, tighten victim's clothing and help victim lean on their back with feet on floor and knees raised.

**First aid for shock**; shock is mainly experienced due to the affinity of nutrients and oxygen that can meet the body's needs. Blood is the main carrier of both blood and nutrients. Blood loss might be the first thing you will notice on a shock victim.

Shock is a life-threatening emergency. There are a number of types of shock namely anaphylactic, cardiogenic and hypovolemic. Anaphylactic involve allergies that cause swelling of air passages preventing the flow of oxygen and a lack of oxygen in the blood. A hypovolemic shock involves a loss of blood from the circulatory system whereas cardiogenic shock is caused by ineffective pumping of blood in the body. This is usually as a result of heart problems and heart attack.

The symptoms of shock include sweating, a pale, cold and clammy skin and a rapid pulse at the first phase. For developing phase of shock, your body shows signs of dizziness, nausea, rapid and shallow breathing, thirst, weak pulse, and cyanosis.

In an advanced phase of developing your body shows an absence of a pulse from the wrist, restlessness, aggressiveness, yawning and unconsciousness. In the final phase, a cardiac arrest may make its appearance.

For a shock, a health care provider checks the carotid pulse of a victim. The victim is first laid in a recovery position. You first need to maintain a victim's blood flow to the head and thorax.

To do this have the victim's body laid flat on the floor and their legs raised about 15-30 cm or 6-12 inches off the ground.

Other significant factors of a shock treatment include Warmth, ABCs, Rest, and Reassurance.

If the patient is unconscious, do the ABCs with a patient at recovery and call an ambulance.

**Asthma and hyperventilation first aid**: asthma is well known as the inflammation of an airway that prevents air exchange. Hyperventilation is breathing at an unreasonably high rate.

Asthma can be noticed in a victim through signs like wheezing, difficulty in breathing, increased airway secretions and an asthma history. For a hyperventilation will involve faster breathing rate and lightheadedness. It can also be described as one not able to catch one's breath.

For an asthma attack advice the victim to go an inhaler, you can help them locate one. Help the victim match your breathing patterns as they lower their rate of breathing.

If the victim has a fast-acting inhaler for asthma attacks, encourage them to use it. You may assist with finding the inhaler. Help victim match your breathing patterns and calm the victim while slowing their breathing rate. Help the casualty sit in a position that relieves pressure on the chest. They can sit in a tripod position; sitting up, leaning slightly forward and supporting their weight with their arms on an object or their knees. Call for emergency medical services if the victim's condition does not improve or if the patient goes unconscious.

For a hyperventilation condition, you need to calm the patient so as to reduce their rate of breathing. You can also increase the amount of carbon dioxide in the air they breathe. You can do this by allowing them breathe into a plastic bag.

First aid for an obstructed airway for conscious and unconscious victims and infants: In the case of conscious victim, you can perform abdominal thrusts; use your hands to exert some pressure below the diaphragm. This act compresses lungs and exerts pressure on the object that was trapped in your trachea having it expelled. This results in a cough.

Even when performed in the right way, this act can injure a person and, therefore, you should encourage them to cough.

You can identify an airway obstruction by signs like a person desperately grabbing their neck, a person not able to speak or even cry out and a person's face turning blue due to a lack of oxygen.

Note that abdominal thrusts are only used on conscious adults and children victims. Before performing the thrusts ask your victim whether they are choking, do not interfere but encourage them to cough.

Perform the thrusts if the condition appears severe by:

- Standing behind the victim and wrapping your arms around a victim's side, below their arms.
- A hand should be in fist form and placed thumb side in, flat against a victim's upper abdomen, below the ribs but above the navel.

- The other hand grabs the fist and directs it upwards in that series of thrusts as the object gets expelled.
- The thrusts should not restrict the ribcage in whatever way.
- If you cannot perform the thrust because of the size of the victim's diaphragm or due to pregnancy, you can perform them at the chest.
- In the case that the victim loses consciousness, call for an ambulance.
- In the case of an infant, a severe obstruction can be accompanied by a high pitched, crow like sound not present in children and adults.

For infants, a severe obstruction may be accompanied by a high-pitched, crow-like sound. This is as a result of the incomplete formation of the infant's airway. Here you need to replace the abdominal thrusts with 5 chest thrusts and 5 back blows.

- First, hold an infant with head in your hand, spine along a forearm and head below the rest of the body.
- Compress the infant's chest 5 times as infant CPR
- Shift infant to the other forearm; chest now against the arm
- Perform 5 back blows with infant's head against below the rest of the body
- Continue till the obstruction is cleared or infant goes unconscious

For an unconscious victim since the airway is shut, you are required to call for emergency medical services. Perform a primary assessment and carry out

CPR to keep your victim alive as you wait for the medics

**First aid for burns**: Burns are soft tissue injuries and come in different degrees of burns. The degrees of burns include superficial burns, full thickness, and partial thickness.

A superficial burn; first degree of burns that exhibits pain, dryness, red and swelled skin, a partial thickness burn is a second degree burn, it exhibits redness, swelling, pain and blisters that when open can release clear fluid. A full thickness burn is a third-degree burn and can destroy underlying tissues like nerves, bones, muscles and fat. For this degree of burn, the skin is black, brown or appears charred. Tissues blow will appear white, painful or at times painless depending on the situation of the nerves.

These burns can be caused heat, chemicals, electricity, and radiation. In the case of a thermal burn, stop the burning by having the person removed from the source of burn. Perform ABCs and cool the burns with some water until the pains are alleviated.

Dress the burn loosely with a sterile non-adhesive dressing. Avoid using creams, butter and oils. These substances can trap heat and even cause an infection. They can also cause pain at the hospital since they will need some cleaning. You should also avoid antiseptics that may irritate sensitive skin. Treat for shock since burns can cripple a body's ability to regulate any kind of heat.

Medications commonly used include an Aloe-Vera extract, Silverdene, Topical Analgesics and NSAIDs like aspirin and ibuprofen. Before any medication consult a doctor for advice.

For a chemical burn do not break blisters, clean a burn, remove a cloth that burned on the wound, apply any ointment, touch a burn with an unsterile covering and apply or iced water.

If the skin has any dry chemical, brush off the skin using a cloth, paper or a gloved hand. Be careful not get any chemical on yourself or the victim. After getting rid of the bulk chemical, flush with running water and call emergency medical services. If the chemical was wet, flush with copious amounts of water as you call the emergency medical services.

Electrical burns resemble third-degree burns. The wounds usually comprise of an entry wound and an exit wound. Call for emergency medical services if the person was shocked. An electrocution can cause cardiac and respiratory complications. Always give care and CPR as you wait for the medics.

Radiation burns resemble thermal burns in their treatment. These burns can be as a result of nuclear or UV radiations. Radiation burns cannot be handled by a lay rescuer. Individuals working in high-risk environments are trained on how to handle this condition. A lay rescuer can risk their self unknowingly by exposing their self to the radiations when treating the victim. For a nuclear radiation, burn call emergency medical services.

Sometimes radiation burns can come in the form of snow-blindness. Cover the victim's eyes with sterile gauze and immediately call emergency medical services.

Keep the victim comfortable, monitor the ABCs, treat shock and keep the victim calm.

For critical burns, immediate medical attention is required. These burns can be disabling, disfiguring and life-threatening. Call EMS if the burns are as a result of chemical or electricity, if burns to a mouth or nose have resulted in a blockage in the airway, if the victim burnt is a child or an elderly person, if the victim has breathing difficulties, if the burns are experienced more than a body part, if the burns affect the head, genitals, necks, hands and the feet.

First aid for electrocution: these are a set of injuries resulting from direct contact with live electric currents. Electrocution can vary and mostly range from a minor injury to a cardiac arrest. Before treating an electrocuted victim, ensure he or she is not in contact with live electricity. Turn off power at the main switch. You can remove the victim from the currents using a wood pole. Be clear from any electric dangers.

Cut any contact with the victim to a live electric source. You can do this with a non-conductive object and even break contact between source and victim.

Call the police and professional rescuers to come and ensure the power lines are not alive. You should also call an ambulance for a case of electrocution. Either the victim is conscious or unconscious; they require assessment at a hospital.

After ensuring the scene is now safe do a primary assessment to check on the ABCs and even begin a CPR if required. Do a secondary assessment to look out for two electric burns. Electric burns resemble third-degree burns; they should be covered by non-stick and sterile dressings.

A victim experiencing a cardiac arrest is more serious than a burn. An electrocution can cause unconsciousness for some time.

A primary assessment will help check the ABCs and if the casualty isn't breathing a CPR begins. An airway can swell as a result of breathing.

For a serious shock do not bother to have the victim at a recovery position. Injuries of the head, the back, and the neck can result from muscle contractions caused by the electrocution. Monitor the cardiac rhythm for disturbances which can cause a cardiac arrest

The electrocution may not cause unconsciousness. Here the victim may feel unwell after the experience and even complain of numbness and a feeling of pins in the area affected by the electrocution. These victims should be transported to the hospital for medication.

**First aid for chest and abdominal injuries**: the injuries experienced in this case involve closed and open chest injuries. The chest protects most of the vital parts of a human body on the upper part. A chest injury should receive professional medical attention. Consider calling an ambulance for any sort of chest injury. Some of these closed chest injuries include broken ribs. This injury can be very painful. A rib fracture has a risk of causing an internal injury like puncturing a lung leading to lung collapsing.

There are a number of rib fracture patterns. Some of these include flail chest which refers to rib fractures along the same rib. This causes a float in the chest segment causing a difficulty in breathing. Another pattern is a stove chest whereby all the ribs have fractured. Here the ribcage loses in rigidness and even a difficulty in breathing.

You can recognize this condition in a victim if he or she shows signs of shallow breathing, trouble breathing, tenderness at injured region, deformity of the chest, and an uneven expansion of the chest, pain upon movement of chest cavity, blood cough, cyanosis and crackling sensation for a punctured lung.

The first aid treatment for these include an ABC assessment, calling an ambulance, having the victim in a position of comfort, conducting a secondary survey and even monitoring the vital carefully.

An open chest wound also known as a chest penetrated by a sharp object, can be recognized by escaping air from that wound, an entrance and exit wound, trouble breathing, a sucking sound as air escapes the chest blood stained bubbles due to an exhalation or even coughing blood.

The treatment will involve ABC assessment, not removing the object, calling an ambulance, flutter valve over the wound, positioning the victim laterally (injured side down), treat shock, have a secondary survey and monitor the vitals.

**Making a flutter valve**

Have a plastic material larger than the wound. Something like a credit card. Tape plastic patch over the wound on three sides with the fourth side left open. This is to allow blood to drain and air to escape. The opening should be at the bottom depending on the victim's position

In the case of an abdominal injury, avoid pushing back victim's organs if the injuries protrude outside the abdominal wall. Have the victim laid flat with the knees bent and covers organs with a moist, sterile dressing; use gauze avoid paper products.

The victim should not drink or eat even with thirst. Call EMS for shock and monitor ABCs until an emergency medical team arrives. If the injury did not result in an open wound, have the victim laid flat with knees bent, treat for a shock as you wait for medics.

A sprain, fracture, bone or joint injuries come with the same symptoms and, therefore, difficult to identify a specific type of injury. However, the treatment is the same for all of them. Some of the symptoms they exhibit include deformity at the injury site, crepitus; grinding or cracking sound in affected area, bruising, swelling, and not able to use a part.

Inform the EMS if the injury turns out to be severe.

The treatment for any joint, muscle, or bone injury follows the mnemonic RICE for rest, immobilize, cold and elevation.

Rest helps soft tissue injuries at short or long-term, immobilization helps strains, sprains, and dislocations. The fractures are slinged and splinted. Cold, C should be used at times for 10 to 20 minutes at a time. To avoid any problems place some fabric between ice and skin. Elevation, E implies that the injury should be elevated to reduce on localized swelling but avoid elevating if pain is caused.

For poisoning the treatment is obtained from accompanying labels or MSDS (Material Safety Data Sheet). You are advised to transport immediately the poisoned victim to advanced medical care like the EMS. The victim first requires basic life support and ABCS at any moment.

Poison gets to one's body through inhalation, injection, absorption, and ingestion pass through the unbroken skin. Absorbed poisons are quite dangerous by not only causing local damage but also widespread damage which is through the blood stream. Some of these chemicals include insecticides and agricultural chemicals.

The treatment is an initial assessment as you call for the EMS. You should carry out any life-threatening problems and move to the removal of the poison.

You can remove the poison in various ways like powders, chemical in the eye and use of some liquids.

You just need to wear a glove, brush powder on victim and irrigate region affected with the copious amount of water for some time. In the case of a liquid, flush with water for about 20 minutes and if the chemical got into your eyes, flush your eyes with clean water for the same amount of time, 20 minutes. Absorbed chemical should be gotten rid of immediately to prevent further damage to a victim's body.

Inhalation injuries can be obtained from smoke, chemicals, and gasses. Get the victim to fresh air and use caution in rescue breathing to avoid getting contaminated.

Ingestion can cause internal poisoning. Vomiting is not a good sign for diagnosis that you are poisoned. A good indication is the presence of an open container of medication or household chemicals. Have a look at the label for any specific first aid instructions.

Call EMS immediately for advanced medical care. You can also call a pest control center and provide information about the poison suspected. This call can help come up with the first aid for this condition.

Another poisoning way is through injection. This ranges from drug abuse to insect sting and bites. A poison control center can provide the best advice for the first aid of this condition.

A basic treatment for this will involve monitoring of the victim's ABCs, dealing with shock, attending to a patient's allergic reactions and calm the patient. To help the medics when they arrive have as much information on the poison as you can. This may entail what it the poison was, when it was injected, how it was injected, and even on whatever allergic reactions the victim has exhibited.

Seizures are as a result of random, uncontrolled electrical activity in the brain. Seizures occur when electrical activities of your brain are irregular. A seizure is a medical emergency. A seizure can be caused by a serious condition like epilepsy.

Some of the risks for seizures include head trauma, brain or spinal infections, epilepsy, stroke, drug use or withdrawal, low blood sugar, heat stroke and fever in infants. Prior to a seizure, there is an aura feeling that normally precedes it. Some of these victims may be aware and inform those around them to stay low prevent injury.

Normally a seizure does not last more than three minutes. Some of its common symptoms include irregular breathing, body rigidness, convulsions, urination, and drooling.

During treatment do not strain the seizure, don't put anything in their mouth, do not hold them to stop the seizure, a tongue may block the airway, but this is normal.

To care for a seizure: call the EMS, move anything that might injure the victim, support victim's head from injury, request bystanders to leave since the person affected may embarrassed after a seizure, if there is no suspicion of spinal injury roll victim to recovery, the victim slowly awakens and ensure bystanders are away to offer reassurance for the victim. The victim will be very tired after a seizure. Reassure the victim until they are fully aware of the surroundings or as they wait for the EMS.

**Head and facial injuries' first aid**: A head wound requires special care due to the possibility of a brain damage. Their treatment is the same as that of a flesh wound. A number of precautions should be taken during this treatment. If the victim's head condition led to a decreased level of consciousness, take the victim to a physician for assessment. This injury also requires an assessment of spinal injury.

There are two known types of a head injury namely a concussion and a compression. A concussion involves a mild head injury that causes a brief short circuit to the brain and rattled skull. There might be no signs of injury to a brain tissue.

A concussion can be noticed by a short period of consciousness, vomiting, visual disturbances i.e.

seeing stars, confusion, memory loss, unequal sized pupils, headaches, anxiety, and agitation.

In the case of a concussion, there is pressure in the brain due to the buildup of fluid, bruised brain, tissue damage. These symptoms worsen over time.

You can recognize this by short term unconsciousness, daze and confusion, visual disturbance, amnesia, pupil unequal in size, head pains, agitation and anxiety and worsening of symptoms over time.

The treatment for these two head injuries includes EMS, immobilization of the spine, treating for any kind of bleeding

Call for medical assistance if the victim's conscious condition changes and avoid using direct pressure for the bleeding if the skull is bruised to avoid compression the injury further.

**Eye injuries first aid**: injuries in eyelid and tissues around the eye need to be handled carefully. If the injury does not involve an eyelid, then apply a sterile compress and hold with a firm bandage. Do not remove any object trapped in the eye. Have the victim lying down as you seek medical attention for this kind of injury. Removal of the objects can result in vision impairment.

As a rescuer do not allow the victim to rub the eye. Any disturbance can result to further harm. Be gentle as you handle this kind of injury. Do not use a sharp object to remove the object. Only trained medical personnel can handle such cases.

Remove small objects by:

Wash the eye with sterile and lukewarm water. Use a sterile medicine dropper or syringe with victim's eye lying towards a side. Direct water to an inside corner of the eye and allow it get rid of the objects towards the outside part of the eye.

If you see, the objects remove with the corner of a clean handkerchief or moist cotton swab. Do not use a dry cloth in getting rid of the object you might hurt the victim and end up not helping out with the situation.

If you do not see the object with the lower lid down, turn the upper lid back and tell the victim to look down and have the applicator lengthwise across the upper lid. Grasp lashes of the upper lid gently but firmly. Pull up on eyelashes turning lid back over the applicator. If you see, the objects use the handkerchief corner. If you cannot remove the object, do not attempt to, hold the eye with small and thick gauze, holding with a loose bandage to limit the movement of the injured eye. Immediately seek medical help for the victim.

**First aid for** heat stroke, heat cramps, and heat exhaustion: a heat cramp is experienced when a person has been active in hot weather and has gotten dehydrated. You can deal with this by taking the person to a shady area, stretch calf and thigh muscles through a cramp, hydrate the victim using lesser salt concentration substances; give the victim a saltine cracker to eat as they drink and have the victim at rest. If cramp continues, seek medical assistance for the victim.

A heat exhaustion occurs after several days of exposure to high temperatures. The victim ends up having an inadequate replacement of fluids. Elderly people with a high blood pressure experience this most. You can also suffer from this by working and working out in a hot environment.

Heat exhaustion is shown by the presence of a headache, nausea and vomiting, fainting, weakness, muscle cramps, fatigue, and paleness. Its treatment can be administered by loosening any tight clothing, applying cool and wet cloths and moving to an aired area. EMS is not required unless the victim experiences a heat stroke.

A heat stroke results from a body beyond its cooling mechanisms. This condition can cause death in just minutes. The symptoms of a heat stroke include unconsciousness, an abnormal mental status, hot and dry skin, dizziness and confusion, higher blood pressure, hyperventilation, a higher temperature of more than 105 degrees F.

To treat, call EMS and cool the victim down. As you do your first aid keep in mind that the higher the body heats, the higher the chances of a victim dying. Use water, apply cold and wet towels. You can pack ice into victim's heat loss areas but do not allow it to be in contact with skin. This can cause frost bite. Have the victim in the coolest area possible, maintain an open airway, expose victim to air condition, give a conscious victim cool water to drink and be ready to give a CPR if the victim goes unconscious.

There are also cold-related conditions that require first aid. These conditions include frostbite and hypothermia. Frostbite involves the freezing of tissues. A skin can freeze more than the skin's depth, a deep frostbite. The treatment for frostbite involves ensuring the skin does not re-freeze after thawing to avoid any more damage, removing victim from a cold region to avoid hypothermia, have the affected part in water which is at a room temperature and skin retaining its condition. Lastly, have the victim taken to a medic for further assessment of the condition.

Hypothermia involves the body temperature dropping beyond its ability to warm itself back. A severe hypothermia is characterized by a body temperature dropping below 95 degrees F. As you treat the victim do not jostle a victim of extreme hypothermia. This may result in a cardiac arrest. Remove victim from cold region, replace any wet cloth on victim with a dry one, use heat pack to treat victim, wrap patient with blanket, and if the victim is conscious advise them to take a warm drink. Call EMS for signs of slurred speech, fumbling hands, confusion and unconsciousness.

Pressure- related illnesses first aid is mainly experienced by divers and swimmers. The weight of water above them can lead to injuries as a result of changes in air pressure. The treatment will involve monitoring of vitals and ABCs, raising victim's legs and feet, bubbles present in bloodstream will move up and prevent any stroke and heart attack, such victims require recompression and, therefore, the need for EMS. If trained in oxygen administration and have equipment administer a higher oxygen flow.

A common condition experienced is bends also known as decompression. As a diver ascends the pressure of water column decreases. The gasses in the blood stream no longer get dissolved in the blood stream and form bubbles. The location of bubbles determines the type of decompression sickness you develops. If they form in the lungs, an air embolism develops.

You can notice this condition in a victim through signs like a symptomatic sensation in the elbows, knees, shoulders, and ankles. These symptoms are well shown in a DCS table.

The last on conditions is the first aid for diabetes. Diabetes is a condition that hampers the regulation of blood sugar (glucose). Insulin allows glucose transmission from the blood stream to cells. The two conditions related to this include hypoglycemia and hyperglycemia.

A hypoglycemia also known as an insulin shock is a condition whereby the blood sugar levels are quite low to power a body. The symptoms appear suddenly and can result from lack of food, excessive exercise, too much insulin and a vomited meal.

You will recognize this condition with the help of symptoms like paleness and clamminess, dizziness and weakness, hunger, seizures, confusion and a strong and rapid pulse. This condition can be confused with a stroke or a cardiac disorder.

The treatment for this condition will include testing glucose level to identify the type of glucose level. Monitor ABCs, if victim is conscious give glucose, treat for shock, advice victim to use their own emergency kit, if the victim carried their insulin injection allow they administer it themselves and seek EMS for an unconscious victim.

Hyperglycemia is a condition whereby the body's blood sugar level is too high to maintain. This is an uncommon and slow condition. Causes of this condition include lesser insulin intake, high glucose intake, and an infection.

You can recognize this condition through symptoms like redness of the skin, loss of appetite, rapid respirations, dehydration, and dizziness, a weak and rapid pulse.

You can handle this condition by monitoring ABCs, treating for shock, encouraging a victim to use a diabetic emergency kit like insulin injections, assist if required and even call EMS.

## Chapter 6: Safety measures during a first aid

As a rescuer, you are also a potential victim to the dangers of a scene. Dangers come in various ways. These dangers include environmental and human dangers. The surroundings that are dangerous to carry out a first aid include falling masonry, broken glass, fast vehicles or chemicals. Human dangers can be caused by people at the scene; accidental or intentional. Some of these devices include:

Your surrounding can be a real source of danger. Always be aware of what is around you and the possible dangers.

Take steps to minimize the risk to yourself. Some of the dangers include body fluids like urine, vomit, feces, and blood. These fluids can cause cross contamination. Other risks they carry include infections and diseases. You, therefore, need barrier devices and other safety equipment.

A common barrier device is a glove. Gloves can be classified as purple nitrile, latex, and vinyl. Gloves will help you away from the risk of fluids like feces, bodily fluids, parasite and dermatological infections. Have gloves on before approaching a victim.

Nitrile gloves are the most expensive but recommended gloves. They are impermeable to body fluids and feces. Material used in their manufacture can deal with chemical spills and burns. You can brush off chemical with this type of glove.

Latex gloves are mainly white gloves. These gloves are most common for allergies and therefore before handling a condition as the victim if they are allergic to latex. Allergies are not life threatening, but it serves right to ask the victim.

Vinyl gloves are at times found in kits. These gloves are advisable for use on victims without an external body fluid because of their high break rate. It will be ok not having them in a kit to avoid confusion.

Another barrier device is the CPR adjunct. This device helps perform a safe mouth-to-mouth resuscitation. A mouth-to-mouth resuscitation keeps you at risk of bodily fluid contact. This is most common for victims with a mouth infections and regurgitated stomach contents. This device has made it easier for anyone to perform a CPR. A CPR can come in the form of small key rings with a nitrile plastic shield or a fitted rescue 'pocket mask' with an oxygen inlet.

A safety glass is also useful equipment during a first aid. This equipment helps prevent any spurting fluid which could spray and come into contact with the eyes.

An apron will help protect rescuers clothing from contamination.

A filter breathing mask filters out harmful chemicals or pathogens. You can use this equipment when handling victim suffering from a communicable respiratory infection like tuberculosis.

Most kits have instructions on how to use the equipment they carry. Sometimes you will not carry a kit with you and, therefore, need to improvise some.

Some of the prevalent improvisations include gloves, gauzes, splints, slings, and stretchers. You can improvise a glove by using dish gloves, plastic bags and leather gloves. Ensure you clean your hands after the usage.

You can make gauze from clean clothing. Avoid the use of paper products.

Have simple splints from straight sections of cardboard, wood, plastic, or metal.

A sling can be made from a victim's clothing.

Improvise a stretcher by using a long and strong clothing, bed sheet, duvet or blanket.

## Conclusion

This book has described all that will help you learn a lot about first aid. The list of emergency and first aid conditions is long but this book has made your journey as a rescuer easy.

Thank you again for downloading this book. I am extremely excited to pass this information along to you and also happy that you now have read it. You can give a try to its guidelines; you will surely enjoy it.

Finally, if you enjoyed this book and feel it has brought a different dimension of thinking about your safety and that of your home and victim. Please take the time to share your thoughts and post a review on Amazon. It'd be greatly appreciated!

Thank you and good luck!

## Disclaimer

Considerable energy has been used to provide the most up to date, accurate, and relative information in this eBook, but the reader is strongly encouraged to seek professional advice prior to using any of this information contained in this eBook. Reader understands that neither the author nor the publisher of this eBook is in any way a professional. The reader also understands they are reading and using this information contained herein at their own risk, and in no way will the author or the publisher be held responsible for any damages whatsoever.

www.ingramcontent.com/pod-product-compliance
Lightning Source LLC
Chambersburg PA
CBHW070130290526
45789CB00005B/2186